JUICING AND SMOOTHIES FOR CHRONIC KIDNEY DISEASE

Kidney friendly fruit blends and vegetable recipes to detox and reduce kidney failure

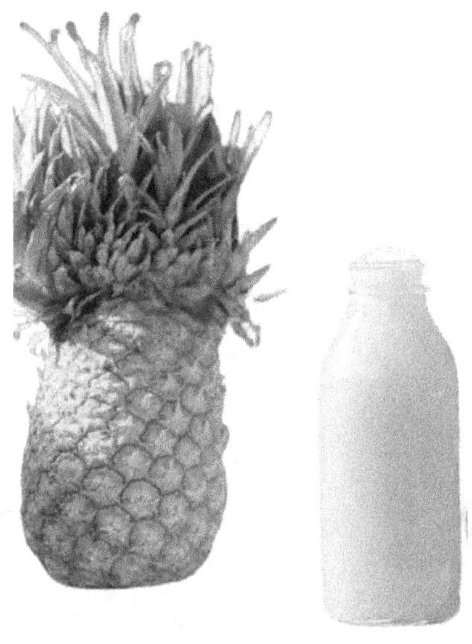

Dr. Malvin Harison

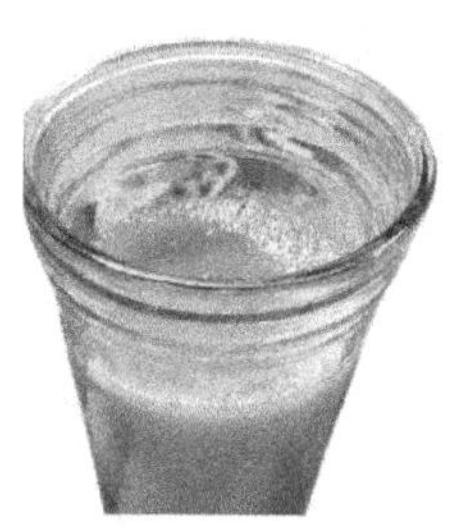

TABLE OF CONTENT

Introduction

A Journey Through Nutrient-Rich Recipes for Chronic Kidney Diseases

In the intricate tapestry of our health, our kidneys stand as silent guardians, orchestrating a delicate balance within our bodies. Yet, for those navigating the challenges of Chronic Kidney Disease (CKD), this symphony can become disrupted, demanding a nuanced approach to nourishment and well-being.

Welcome to "Renewed Vitality," a collection of nutrient-rich recipes tailored to support individuals on their journey through Chronic Kidney Disease.

This book serves as a gateway to understanding the intricacies of nutrition for those living with CKD.
It unveils a world where vibrant fruits, wholesome grains, and nourishing

proteins converge to create meals that are both palate-pleasing and kidney-friendly. From antioxidant-rich berries to low-phosphorus grains, each ingredient is selected with care, bearing in mind its potential impact on kidney function.

So, let the aroma of wholesome ingredients fill your kitchen as you delve into this culinary voyage. May each dish be a step towards renewed vitality, a celebration of life's flavors in harmony with the intricate needs of your kidneys. Here's to "Renewed Vitality"—a guide, a companion, and a flavorful pathway towards well-being for those navigating the landscape of Chronic Kidney Disease.

Understanding the term ''Chronic Kidney Disease ''

Chronic Kidney Disease (CKD) is a persistent condition marked by a gradual decline in kidney function over time. The kidneys, vital for filtering waste and regulating bodily functions, lose their efficiency. CKD is categorized into stages, from mild to severe, based on the kidneys' filtration rate. Causes include diabetes, high blood pressure, and genetic factors.

Symptoms may be subtle initially but can progress to fatigue, swelling, and changes in urine output. Management involves lifestyle changes, medications, and, in severe cases, dialysis or transplantation. A kidney-friendly diet, controlling nutrients like sodium and potassium, is crucial.
Regular monitoring by healthcare professionals is vital for effective management and improved outcomes. Early detection is key in addressing Chronic Kidney Disease.

Stages of Chronic Kidney Disease

Chronic Kidney Disease (CKD) is divided into stages based on the estimated Glomerular Filtration Rate (eGFR), which measures the kidneys' ability to filter blood. The stages range from 1 to 5:

1. Stage 1: Kidney Damage
- eGFR is normal or slightly increased.
- Evidence of kidney damage, such as protein in the urine (albuminuria).

2. Stage 2: Mild Reduction in Function
- Slight decrease in eGFR.
- Kidney damage is more apparent.

3. Stage 3: Moderate Reduction in Function
- Further decrease in eGFR.
- Kidney function is noticeably impaired.
- Subdivided into 3A (mild to moderate) and 3B (moderate to severe).

4. Stage 4: Severe Reduction in Function

- Significant decline in eGFR.
- Kidney function is severely compromised.
- Subdivided into 4A (severe) and 4B (very severe).

5. Stage 5: End-Stage Renal Disease (ESRD)

- eGFR is extremely low.
- Kidneys are no longer able to function adequately to sustain life.
- Dialysis or kidney transplantation is usually necessary.

Importance of taking the right diet to the disease

Adopting the right diet is paramount for individuals with chronic diseases like Chronic Kidney Disease (CKD). The significance of a proper diet lies in its ability to positively impact overall health, slow disease progression, and manage symptoms. Conversely, neglecting dietary guidelines can lead to complications and exacerbate the challenges associated with the disease.

Importance of the Right Diet:

1. Managing Symptoms: A well-balanced diet helps control symptoms such as fluid retention, high blood pressure, and electrolyte imbalances commonly associated with CKD.

2. Slowing Progression: Following a kidney-friendly diet can slow the progression of CKD,
preserving kidney function and delaying the need for more aggressive interventions like dialysis or transplantation.

3. Nutrient Control: Controlling intake of key nutrients like sodium, potassium, and phosphorus is crucial in preventing imbalances that can strain the kidneys and worsen the disease.

4. Blood Pressure Regulation: A heart-healthy diet aids in regulating blood pressure, a crucial factor in CKD management as hypertension is both a cause and a consequence of kidney disease.

5. Minimizing Complications: Proper nutrition supports the management of related conditions, such as diabetes, which often coexists with CKD.

Complications of Neglecting the Right Diet

1. Fluid Overload: Inadequate fluid control can lead to fluid retention, causing swelling and increasing the risk of high blood pressure and heart-related complications.

2. Electrolyte Imbalances: Failure to regulate sodium and potassium intake can result in electrolyte imbalances, affecting nerve and muscle function and potentially leading to life-threatening complications.

3. Worsened Kidney Function: High-protein diets or excessive intake of certain nutrients can strain the kidneys, accelerating the decline in kidney function.

4. Cardiovascular Risks: Poor diet choices contribute to cardiovascular issues, which are a leading cause of mortality in individuals with CKD.

5. Bone Health: Imbalances in phosphorus and calcium can affect bone health, leading to conditions like renal osteodystrophy.

6. Increased Fatigue: Malnutrition resulting from an inadequate diet can contribute to fatigue and reduced overall well-being.

Foods to Eat for Chronic Kidney Disease (CKD)

1. Low-Potassium Fruits
- Apples
- Berries (strawberries, blueberries)
- Pineapple
- Watermelon (in moderation)

2. Low-Phosphorus Vegetables
- Cauliflower
- Cabbage
- Bell peppers
- Radishes

3. Lean Proteins
- Skinless poultry
- Fish (salmon, trout)
- Eggs
- Low-fat dairy (milk, yogurt)

4. Low-Sodium Grains

- White bread
- White rice
- Pasta
- Cereal (low-sodium)

5. Heart-Healthy Fats
- Olive oil
- Avocado
- Nuts (in moderation)
- Flaxseeds

6. Low-Fluid Fruits
- Grapes
- Peaches
- Cranberries
- Applesauce

7. Herbs and Spices
- Parsley
- Basil
- Cilantro
- Garlic (in moderation)

8. Berries

- Blueberries
- Raspberries
- Strawberries
- Cranberries

Foods to Avoid or Limit for Chronic Kidney Disease

1. High-Potassium Foods
- Bananas
- Oranges
- Potatoes
- Tomatoes and tomato products

2. High-Phosphorus Foods
- Dairy products (hard cheeses, milk)
- Nuts and seeds
- Whole grains
- Chocolate

3. High-Sodium Foods
- Processed foods
- Canned soups and broths
- Pickled foods
- Deli meats

4. High-Protein Foods
- Red meat
- Processed meats (sausages, bacon)
- Organ meats (liver, kidney)
- Full-fat dairy

5. High-Fluid Foods
   - Soups with high water content
   - Ice cream
   - Gelatin desserts
   - Watery fruits (watermelon in excess)

6. Certain Vegetables
   - Spinach
   - Swiss chard
   - Beets
   - Potatoes (if not properly leached)

7. Excessive Sugar
   - Sugary snacks
   - Soda and sugary drinks
   - High-sugar desserts

8. Alcohol
   - Limit alcohol intake, as it can contribute to dehydration and affect kidney function.

Chapter 1: Nutritious Juicing Recipes For Chronic Kidney Disease

Here are juicing recipes tailored for individuals with Chronic Kidney Disease:

1. Cucumber-Mint Cooler

Ingredients

- 1 cucumber
- A handful of mint leaves
- 1 green apple
- 1/2 lemon (peeled)

Instructions

1. Wash all ingredients thoroughly.
2. Cut them into small pieces.
3. Juice the cucumber, mint, apple, and lemon.
4. Mix well and serve over ice.

Servings: 1

Nutritional Value (per serving)

- Calories: 50
- Vitamin K

- Hydration support

2. Carrot-Orange Delight

Ingredients
- 3 carrots
- 2 oranges (peeled)
- 1/2 inch ginger

Instructions
1. Peel and chop carrots.
2. Peel oranges.
3. Juice carrots, oranges, and ginger.
4. Stir well and serve chilled.

Servings: 1

Nutritional Value (per serving)
- Calories: 120
- Vitamin A
- Antioxidants

3. Pineapple-Kale Elixir

Ingredients
- 1 cup pineapple chunks
- 1 cup kale leaves
- 1 green apple
- 1/2 lemon (peeled)

Instructions

1. Prepare pineapple, kale, apple, and lemon.
2. Juice all ingredients.
3. Mix thoroughly and serve over ice.

Servings: 1

Nutritional Value (per serving)

- Calories: 100
- Vitamin C
- Iron

4. Berry-Basil Refresher

Ingredients

- 1/2 cup blueberries
- 1/2 cup strawberries
- 1/2 cup raspberries
- A handful of basil leaves

Instructions

1. Wash berries and basil leaves.
2. Juice all ingredients together.
3. Stir well and enjoy.

Servings: 1

Nutritional Value (per serving)

- Calories: 60
- Fiber

- Antioxidants

5. Apple-Celery Cleanse

Ingredients
- 2 green apples
- 4 celery stalks
- 1/2 cucumber
- 1/2 lemon (peeled)

Instructions
1. Clean and chop apples, celery, cucumber, and lemon.
2. Juice all ingredients.
3. Mix well and serve chilled.

Servings: 1

Nutritional Value (per serving)
- Calories: 80
- Hydration support
- Vitamin K

6. Watermelon-Mint Hydrator

Ingredients
- 2 cups watermelon chunks
- A handful of mint leaves
- 1/2 lime (peeled)

Instructions

1. Cube watermelon.

2. Juice watermelon, mint, and lime.

3. Stir and serve over ice.

Servings: 1

Nutritional Value (per serving)

- Calories: 90

- Hydration support

- Vitamin C

7. Ginger-Turmeric Immunity Boost

Ingredients

- 1 inch ginger

- 1/2 inch turmeric

- 2 oranges (peeled)

- 1/2 lemon (peeled)

Instructions

1. Peel and chop ginger and turmeric.

2. Juice ginger, turmeric, oranges, and lemon.

3. Mix well and serve.

Servings: 1

Nutritional Value (per serving)

- Calories: 70

- Anti-inflammatory properties

- Vitamin C

8. Beet-Berry Detoxifier

Ingredients
- 1 medium-sized beetroot
- 1/2 cup blackberries
- 1/2 cup strawberries
- 1/2 lemon (peeled)

Instructions
1. Peel and chop beetroot.
2. Wash berries and peel lemon.
3. Juice all ingredients together.
4. Stir and serve.

Servings: 1

Nutritional Value (per serving)
- Calories: 80
- Detoxifying properties
- Antioxidants

9. Kiwi-Parsley Cleanser

Ingredients
- 2 kiwis
- A handful of parsley
- 1 green apple

- 1/2 lime (peeled)

Instructions

1. Peel and chop kiwis, apple, and lime.
2. Wash parsley.
3. Juice all ingredients.
4. Mix thoroughly and serve chilled.

Servings: 1

Nutritional Value (per serving)

- Calories: 90
- Vitamin K
- Detoxifying properties

10. Mango-Coconut Bliss

Ingredients

- 1 ripe mango
- 1/2 cup coconut water
- A handful of spinach
- 1/2 lime (peeled)

Instructions

1. Peel and chop mango.
2. Juice mango, coconut water, spinach, and lime.
3. Stir well and enjoy.

Servings: 1

Nutritional Value (per serving)

- Calories: 100
- Vitamin C
- Hydration support

11. Cherry-Almond Delight

Ingredients
- 1 cup cherries (pitted)
- 1/2 cup almonds (soaked)
- 1/2 cup cranberries
- 1/2 lime (peeled)

Instructions
1. Wash cherries and cranberries.
2. Soak almonds overnight and drain.
3. Juice cherries, soaked almonds, cranberries, and lime.
4. Mix well and serve over ice.

Servings: 1
Nutritional Value (per serving)
- Calories: 120
- Fiber
- Antioxidants

12. Papaya-Lime Cooler

Ingredients

- 1 cup papaya chunks
- 1/2 lime (peeled)
- A handful of mint leaves
- 1/2 cup coconut water

Instructions

1. Cube papaya.
2. Juice papaya, lime, mint, and coconut water.
3. Stir well and serve chilled.

Servings: 1

Nutritional Value (per serving)

- Calories: 90
- Vitamin C
- Hydration support

13. Pear-Spinach Refresher

Ingredients

- 2 ripe pears
- 1 cup spinach leaves
- 1/2 cucumber
- 1/2 lemon (peeled)

Instructions

1. Peel and chop pears and cucumber.
2. Wash spinach leaves.
3. Juice pears, spinach, cucumber, and lemon.
4. Mix thoroughly and serve over ice.
Servings: 1
Nutritional Value (per serving)
- Calories: 80
- Vitamin K
- Fiber

14. Orange-Ginger Zinger

Ingredients
- 3 oranges (peeled)
- 1 inch ginger
- 1/2 turmeric (optional)
- 1/2 lemon (peeled)

Instructions
1. Peel oranges and chop ginger.
2. Juice oranges, ginger, turmeric, and lemon.
3. Stir well and serve.
Servings: 1
Nutritional Value (per serving)
- Calories: 90

- Anti-inflammatory properties
- Vitamin C

15. Melon-Mint Hydrator

Ingredients
- 1 cup cantaloupe chunks
- 1/2 cup honeydew melon
- A handful of mint leaves
- 1/2 lime (peeled)

Instructions
1. Cube cantaloupe and honeydew melon.
2. Juice melons, mint, and lime.
3. Mix and serve over ice.

Servings: 1

Nutritional Value (per serving)
- Calories: 80
- Vitamin C
- Hydration support

16. Blueberry-Coconut Elixir

Ingredients
- 1 cup blueberries
- 1/2 cup coconut water

- 1/2 cup cucumber
- 1/2 lime (peeled)

Instructions

1. Wash blueberries and cucumber.
2. Juice blueberries, coconut water, cucumber, and lime.
3. Stir well and serve chilled.

Servings 1

Nutritional Value (per serving)

- Calories: 70
- Antioxidants
- Hydration support

17. Avocado-Kale Revitalizer

Ingredients

- 1/2 avocado
- 1 cup kale leaves
- 1 green apple
- 1/2 lemon (peeled)

Instructions

1. Peel and chop avocado, apple, and lemon.
2. Wash kale leaves.
3. Juice all ingredients.
4. Mix thoroughly and serve over ice.

Servings: 1
Nutritional Value (per serving)
- Calories: 100
- Healthy fats
- Vitamin K

18. Blackberry-Beet Elevation

Ingredients
- 1/2 cup blackberries
- 1 medium-sized beetroot
- 1/2 cucumber
- 1/2 lime (peeled)

Instructions
1. Wash blackberries and beetroot.
2. Peel and chop beetroot and cucumber.
3. Juice all ingredients together.
4. Stir and serve over ice.

Servings: 1
Nutritional Value (per serving)
- Calories: 80
- Detoxifying properties
- Antioxidants

19. Tomato-Basil Vitality

Ingredients

- 2 tomatoes
- A handful of basil leaves
- 1/2 cucumber
- 1/2 lime (peeled)

Instructions

1. Wash tomatoes, basil, and cucumber.
2. Peel and chop cucumber.
3. Juice tomatoes, basil, cucumber, and lime.
4. Stir and serve chilled.

Servings: 1

Nutritional Value (per serving)

- Calories: 60
- Vitamin K
- Antioxidants

20. Strawberry-Parsley Cooler

Ingredients

- 1 cup strawberries
- A handful of parsley
- 1/2 cucumber
- 1/2 lemon (peeled)

Instructions

1. Wash strawberries, parsley, and cucumber.
2. Peel and chop cucumber.
3. Juice all ingredients together.
4. Mix well and serve over ice.

Servings: 1

Nutritional Value (per serving)

- Calories: 70
- Vitamin K
- Antioxidants

21. Mango-Basil Bliss

Ingredients

- 1 ripe mango
- A handful of basil leaves
- 1/2 cup pineapple chunks
- 1/2 lime (peeled)

Instructions

1. Peel and chop mango.
2. Wash basil leaves.
3. Juice mango, basil, pineapple, and lime.
4. Mix well and serve chilled.

Servings: 1

Nutritional Value (per serving)
- Calories: 100
- Vitamin C
- Antioxidants

22. Raspberry-Coconut Refresher

Ingredients
- 1/2 cup raspberries
- 1/2 cup coconut water
- 1/2 cucumber
- 1/2 lemon (peeled)

Instructions

1. Wash raspberries and cucumbers.

2. Juice raspberries, coconut water, cucumber, and lemon.

3. Stir well and serve over ice.

Servings: 1

Nutritional Value (per serving)
- Calories: 70
- Antioxidants
- Hydration support

23. Cantaloupe-Celery Soother

Ingredients
- 1 cup cantaloupe chunks
- 3 celery stalks
- 1/2 lime (peeled)
- A pinch of sea salt

Instructions
1. Cube cantaloupe.
2. Wash celery stalks.
3. Juice cantaloupe, celery, lime, and add a pinch of sea salt.
4. Mix thoroughly and serve over ice.

Servings: 1

Nutritional Value (per serving)
- Calories: 80
- Hydration support
- Vitamin C

24. Kiwi-Spinach Rejuvenator

Ingredients
- 2 kiwis
- 1 cup spinach leaves
- 1/2 cucumber
- 1/2 lime (peeled)

Instructions

1. Peel and chop kiwis, cucumber, and lime.

2. Wash spinach leaves.

3. Juice all ingredients together.

4. Mix thoroughly and serve chilled.

Servings: 1

Nutritional Value (per serving)

- Calories: 80

- Vitamin K

- Antioxidants

25. Pomegranate-Parsley Detox

Ingredients

- 1/2 cup pomegranate seeds

- A handful of parsley

- 1/2 cucumber

- 1/2 lemon (peeled)

Instructions

1. Wash pomegranate seeds, parsley, and cucumber.

2. Peel and chop cucumber.

3. Juice all ingredients together.

4. Stir and serve over ice.

Servings: 1
Nutritional Value (per serving)
- Calories: 70
- Detoxifying properties
- Antioxidants

26. Peach-Almond Cooler

Ingredients
- 2 peaches
- 1/2 cup almonds (soaked)
- 1/2 cup coconut water
- 1/2 lime (peeled)
Instructions
1. Wash and pit peaches.
2. Soak almonds overnight and drain.
3. Juice peaches, soaked almonds, coconut water, and lime.
4. Mix well and serve chilled.
Servings: 1
Nutritional Value (per serving)
- Calories: 110
- Fiber
- Healthy fats

27. Blueberry-Beetroot Elevation

Ingredients
- 1/2 cup blueberries
- 1 medium-sized beetroot
- 1/2 cup cucumber
- 1/2 lemon (peeled)

Instructions
1. Wash blueberries and beetroot.
2. Peel and chop beetroot and cucumber.
3. Juice all ingredients together.
4. Stir and serve over ice.

Servings: 1

Nutritional Value (per serving)
- Calories: 80
- Detoxifying properties
- Antioxidants

28. Minty Watermelon Splash

Ingredients
- 2 cups watermelon chunks
- A handful of mint leaves
- 1/2 lime (peeled)

Instructions
1. Cube watermelon.

2. Juice watermelon, mint, and lime.

3. Stir and serve over ice.

Servings: 1

Nutritional Value (per serving)

- Calories: 90

- Hydration support

- Vitamin C

29. Apricot-Ginger Energizer

Ingredients

- 2 apricots

- 1 inch ginger

- 1/2 lime (peeled)

- 1/2 cup coconut water

Instructions

1. Wash and pit apricots.

2. Peel and chop ginger.

3. Juice apricots, ginger, lime, and coconut water.

4. Mix well and serve chilled.

Servings: 1

Nutritional Value (per serving)

- Calories: 70

- Vitamin C

- Hydration support

30. Papaya-Coconut Paradise

Ingredients

- 1 cup papaya chunks
- 1/2 cup coconut water
- A handful of basil leaves
- 1/2 lime (peeled)

Instructions

1. Cube papaya.
2. Juice papaya, coconut water, basil, and lime
3. Mix and serve chilled.

Servings: 1

Nutritional Value (per serving)

- Calories: 90
- Vitamin C
- Antioxidants

Chapter 2: Smoothie recipes for Chronic kidney Disease

Here are smoothie recipes tailored for individuals with Chronic Kidney Disease. These smoothies incorporate kidney-friendly ingredients to support overall health.

1. Berry Blast Smoothie

Ingredients

- 1/2 cup blueberries
- 1/2 cup strawberries
- 1/2 cup raspberries
- 1/2 cup Greek yogurt (low-fat)
- 1/2 banana
- 1 tablespoon chia seeds

Instructions

1. Blend blueberries, strawberries, raspberries, Greek yogurt, banana, and chia seeds until smooth.

2. Pour into a glass and enjoy.

Servings: 1
Nutritional Value (per serving)
- Calories: 150
- Fiber
- Protein

2. Avocado Spinach Smoothie

Ingredients
- 1/2 avocado
- 1 cup spinach leaves
- 1/2 cup cucumber
- 1/2 cup almond milk (unsweetened)
- 1/2 lime (peeled)

Instructions

1. Blend avocado, spinach, cucumber, almond milk, and lime until smooth.

2. Pour into a glass and serve chilled.

Servings: 1
Nutritional Value (per serving)
- Calories: 120
- Healthy fats
- Vitamin K

3. Pineapple Kiwi Delight

Ingredients

- 1 cup pineapple chunks
- 2 kiwis
- 1/2 cup coconut water
- 1/2 cup Greek yogurt (low-fat)

Instructions

1. Blend pineapple, kiwis, coconut water, and Greek yogurt until smooth.
2. Pour into a glass and enjoy.

Servings: 1

Nutritional Value (per serving)

- Calories: 140
- Vitamin C
- Probiotics

4. Cinnamon Apple Smoothie

Ingredients

- 2 apples (peeled and chopped)
- 1/2 teaspoon cinnamon
- 1/2 cup almond milk (unsweetened)
- 1/2 cup Greek yogurt (low-fat)
- 1 tablespoon flax seeds

Instructions

1. Blend apples, cinnamon, almond milk, Greek yogurt, and flaxseeds until smooth.

2. Pour into a glass and serve.

Servings: 1

Nutritional Value (per serving)

- Calories: 180
- Fiber
- Calcium

5. Mango Banana Dream

Ingredients

- 1 ripe mango
- 1/2 banana
- 1/2 cup coconut water
- 1/2 cup Greek yogurt (low-fat)
- 1 tablespoon hemp seeds

Instructions

1. Blend mango, banana, coconut water, Greek yogurt, and hemp seeds until smooth.

2. Pour into a glass and enjoy.

Servings: 1

Nutritional Value (per serving)

- Calories: 160
- Vitamin C
- Protein

6. Strawberry Almond Bliss

Ingredients
- 1 cup strawberries
- 1/2 cup almonds (soaked)
- 1/2 cup almond milk (unsweetened)
- 1/2 cup Greek yogurt (low-fat)
- 1/2 teaspoon vanilla extract

Instructions
1. Blend strawberries, soaked almonds, almond milk, Greek yogurt, and vanilla extract until smooth.
2. Pour into a glass and serve chilled.

Servings: 1

Nutritional Value (per serving)
- Calories: 200
- Fiber
- Protein

7. Peach Mint Refresher

Ingredients

- 2 peaches (peeled and pitted)
- A handful of mint leaves
- 1/2 cup coconut water
- 1/2 cup Greek yogurt (low-fat)

Instructions

1. Blend peaches, mint leaves, coconut water, and Greek yogurt until smooth.
2. Pour into a glass and enjoy.

Servings: 1

Nutritional Value (per serving)

- Calories: 150
- Vitamin C
- Probiotics

8. Cherry Chocolate Smoothie

Ingredients

- 1/2 cup cherries (pitted)
- 1 tablespoon cocoa powder (unsweetened)
- 1/2 cup almond milk (unsweetened)
- 1/2 cup Greek yogurt (low-fat)
- 1 tablespoon chia seeds

Instructions

1. Blend cherries, cocoa powder, almond milk, Greek yogurt, and chia seeds until smooth.

2. Pour into a glass and serve.

Servings: 1

Nutritional Value (per serving)

- Calories: 170
- Fiber
- Protein

9. Raspberry Coconut Smoothie

Ingredients

- 1/2 cup raspberries
- 1/2 cup coconut milk (unsweetened)
- 1/2 cup Greek yogurt (low-fat)
- 1/2 banana
- 1 tablespoon flax seeds

Instructions

1. Blend raspberries, coconut milk, Greek yogurt, banana, and flaxseeds until smooth.

2. Pour into a glass and enjoy.

Servings: 1

Nutritional Value (per serving)

- Calories: 140
- Fiber
- Probiotics

10. Vanilla Berry Protein Smoothie

Ingredients

- 1/2 cup mixed berries (blueberries, strawberries, raspberries)
- 1/2 cup almond milk (unsweetened)
- 1/2 cup Greek yogurt (low-fat)
- 1/2 teaspoon vanilla extract
- 1 scoop protein powder (unflavored)

Instructions

1. Blend mixed berries, almond milk, Greek yogurt, vanilla extract, and protein powder until smooth.
2. Pour into a glass and serve.

Servings: 1

Nutritional Value (per serving)

- Calories: 180
- Protein
- Antioxidants

11. Coconut-Berry Bliss

Ingredients
- 1/2 cup mixed berries (blueberries, strawberries, raspberries)
- 1/2 cup coconut water
- 1/2 cup Greek yogurt (low-fat)
- 1/2 banana
- 1 tablespoon chia seeds

Instructions
1. Blend mixed berries, coconut water, Greek yogurt, banana, and chia seeds until smooth.
2. Pour into a glass and enjoy.

Servings: 1
Nutritional Value (per serving)
- Calories: 160
- Fiber
- Probiotics

12. Orange Carrot Refuel

Ingredients
- 2 oranges (peeled)
- 1/2 cup carrots (chopped)
- 1/2 cup almond milk (unsweetened)

- 1/2 cup Greek yogurt (low-fat)

Instructions

1. Blend oranges, carrots, almond milk, and Greek yogurt until smooth.

2. Pour into a glass and serve chilled.

Servings: 1

Nutritional Value (per serving)

- Calories: 140
- Vitamin C
- Calcium

13. Minty Pineapple Green

Ingredients

- 1 cup pineapple chunks
- A handful of mint leaves
- 1/2 cup spinach leaves
- 1/2 cup coconut water
- 1/2 lime (peeled)

Instructions

1. Blend pineapple, mint leaves, spinach, coconut water, and lime until smooth.

2. Pour into a glass and enjoy.

Servings: 1

Nutritional Value (per serving)

- Calories: 120

- Vitamin C
- Iron

14. Almond Butter Banana Boost

Ingredients
- 1/2 banana
- 1 tablespoon almond butter
- 1/2 cup almond milk (unsweetened)
- 1/2 cup Greek yogurt (low-fat)
- 1/2 teaspoon cinnamon

Instructions
1. Blend banana, almond butter, almond milk, Greek yogurt, and cinnamon until smooth.
2. Pour into a glass and serve.

Servings: 1

Nutritional Value (per serving)
- Calories: 180
- Protein
- Healthy fats

15. Papaya-Coconut Energizer

Ingredients

- 1 cup papaya chunks
- 1/2 cup coconut water
- 1/2 cup Greek yogurt (low-fat)
- 1/2 lime (peeled)
- 1 tablespoon flax seeds

Instructions

1. Blend papaya, coconut water, Greek yogurt, lime, and flaxseeds until smooth.
2. Pour into a glass and enjoy.

Servings: 1

Nutritional Value (per serving)

- Calories: 150
- Vitamin C
- Fiber

16. Peach Basil Infusion

Ingredients

- 2 peaches (peeled and pitted)
- A handful of basil leaves
- 1/2 cup coconut water
- 1/2 cup Greek yogurt (low-fat)

Instructions
1. Blend peaches, basil leaves, coconut water, and Greek yogurt until smooth.
2. Pour into a glass and serve chilled.
Servings: 1
Nutritional Value (per serving)
- Calories: 140
- Vitamin C
- Probiotics

17. Turmeric Mango Lassi

Ingredients
- 1 ripe mango
- 1/2 cup Greek yogurt (low-fat)
- 1/2 teaspoon turmeric
- 1/2 cup almond milk (unsweetened)
Instructions
1. Peel and chop mango.
2. Blend mango, Greek yogurt, turmeric, and almond milk until smooth.
3. Pour into a glass and enjoy.
Servings: 1
Nutritional Value (per serving)
- Calories: 150
- Vitamin C

- Anti-inflammatory properties

18. Kiwi Kale Power Smoothie

Ingredients
- 2 kiwis
- 1 cup kale leaves
- 1/2 cup coconut water
- 1/2 banana
- 1 tablespoon chia seeds

Instructions
1. Peel and chop kiwis.
2. Wash kale leaves.
3. Blend kiwis, kale, coconut water, banana, and chia seeds until smooth.
4. Pour into a glass and serve.

Servings: 1

Nutritional Value (per serving)
- Calories: 130
- Vitamin K
- Fiber

19. Strawberry Oatmeal Smoothie

Ingredients
- 1 cup strawberries
- 1/4 cup rolled oats
- 1/2 cup almond milk (unsweetened)
- 1/2 cup Greek yogurt (low-fat)
- 1 tablespoon honey (optional)

Instructions
1. Blend strawberries, rolled oats, almond milk, Greek yogurt, and honey until smooth.
2. Pour into a glass and enjoy.

Servings: 1

Nutritional Value (per serving)
- Calories: 160
- Fiber
- Protein

20. Blueberry Almond Joy

Ingredients
- 1/2 cup blueberries
- 1/2 cup almonds (soaked)
- 1/2 cup almond milk (unsweetened)
- 1/2 cup Greek yogurt (low-fat)

- 1/2 teaspoon vanilla extract

Instructions

1. Blend blueberries, soaked almonds, almond milk, Greek yogurt, and vanilla extract until smooth.

2. Pour into a glass and serve chilled.

Servings: 1

Nutritional Value (per serving)

- Calories: 190
- Fiber
- Healthy fats

21. Mango Spinach Sunshine

Ingredients

- 1 ripe mango
- 1 cup spinach leaves
- 1/2 cup coconut water
- 1/2 cup Greek yogurt (low-fat)
- 1/2 lime (peeled)

Instructions

1. Peel and chop mango.

2. Wash spinach leaves.

3. Blend mango, spinach, coconut water, Greek yogurt, and lime until smooth.

4. Pour into a glass and serve chilled.

Servings: 1
Nutritional Value (per serving)
- Calories: 140
- Vitamin C
- Iron

22. Raspberry Walnut Refuel

Ingredients
- 1/2 cup raspberries
- 1/2 cup walnuts (soaked)
- 1/2 cup almond milk (unsweetened)
- 1/2 cup Greek yogurt (low-fat)
Instructions
1. Wash raspberries.
2. Soak walnuts overnight and drain.
3. Blend raspberries, soaked walnuts, almond milk, and Greek yogurt until smooth.
4. Pour into a glass and enjoy.
Servings: 1
Nutritional Value (per serving)
- Calories: 200
- Fiber
- Protein

23. Pineapple Mint Fusion

Ingredients

- 1 cup pineapple chunks
- A handful of mint leaves
- 1/2 cup coconut water
- 1/2 cup Greek yogurt (low-fat)

Instructions

1. Blend pineapple, mint leaves, coconut water, and Greek yogurt until smooth.
2. Pour into a glass and serve chilled.

Servings: 1

Nutritional Value (per serving)

- Calories: 130
- Vitamin C
- Probiotics

24. Banana Chia Energizer

Ingredients

- 1/2 banana
- 1 tablespoon chia seeds
- 1/2 cup almond milk (unsweetened)
- 1/2 cup Greek yogurt (low-fat)
- 1/2 teaspoon cinnamon

Instructions

1. Blend banana, chia seeds, almond milk, Greek yogurt, and cinnamon until smooth.

2. Pour into a glass and enjoy.

Servings: 1

Nutritional Value (per serving)

- Calories: 160
- Fiber
- Protein

25. Cucumber Kale Cooler

Ingredients

- 1/2 cucumber
- 1 cup kale leaves
- 1/2 cup coconut water
- 1/2 lime (peeled)

Instructions

1. Wash cucumber and kale leaves.

2. Peel and chop cucumber.

3. Blend cucumber, kale, coconut water, and lime until smooth.

4. Pour into a glass and serve over ice.

Servings: 1

Nutritional Value (per serving)

- Calories: 70
- Vitamin K
- Hydration support

26. Cherry Almond Joy

Ingredients

- 1/2 cup cherries (pitted)
- 1/2 cup almonds (soaked)
- 1/2 cup coconut water
- 1/2 cup Greek yogurt (low-fat)

Instructions

1. Wash cherries.
2. Soak almonds overnight and drain.
3. Blend cherries, soaked almonds, coconut water, and Greek yogurt until smooth.
4. Pour into a glass and serve chilled.

Servings: 1

Nutritional Value (per serving)

- Calories: 180
- Fiber
- Protein

27. Apricot Almond Dream

Ingredients
- 2 apricots
- 1/2 cup almonds (soaked)
- 1/2 cup almond milk (unsweetened)
- 1/2 cup Greek yogurt (low-fat)

Instructions
1. Wash and pit apricots.
2. Soak almonds overnight and drain.
3. Blend apricots, soaked almonds, almond milk, and Greek yogurt until smooth.
4. Pour into a glass and serve.

Servings: 1

Nutritional Value (per serving)
- Calories: 160
- Fiber
- Protein

28. Turmeric Pineapple Twist

Ingredients
- 1 cup pineapple chunks
- 1/2 teaspoon turmeric
- 1/2 cup coconut water

- 1/2 cup Greek yogurt (low-fat)

Instructions

1. Blend pineapple, turmeric, coconut water, and Greek yogurt until smooth.

2. Pour into a glass and serve chilled.

Servings: 1

Nutritional Value (per serving)

- Calories: 140
- Vitamin C
- Anti-inflammatory properties

29. Blueberry Walnut Wonder

Ingredients

- 1/2 cup blueberries
- 1/2 cup walnuts (soaked)
- 1/2 cup almond milk (unsweetened)
- 1/2 cup Greek yogurt (low-fat)

Instructions

1. Wash blueberries.

2. Soak walnuts overnight and drain.

3. Blend blueberries, soaked walnuts, almond milk, and Greek yogurt until smooth.

4. Pour into a glass and enjoy.

Servings: 1

Nutritional Value (per serving)

- Calories: 210
- Fiber
- Protein

30. Minty Melon

Ingredients

- 1 cup cantaloupe chunks
- 1/2 cup honeydew melon
- A handful of mint leaves
- 1/2 lime (peeled)

Instructions

1. Cube cantaloupe and honeydew melon.
2. Wash mint leaves.
3. Blend melons, mint, and lime until smooth.
4. Pour into a glass and serve over ice.

Servings: 1

Nutritional Value (per serving)

- Calories: 90
- Vitamin C
- Hydration support

Conclusion

We've embarked on a journey toward promoting kidney health through a delectable array of smoothies and juices tailored for those managing Chronic Kidney Disease. Remember, the essence of good health lies not only in the foods we choose but in the joy and satisfaction they bring to our lives.

Embrace these recipes as a stepping stone to a kidney-friendly lifestyle, enriched with flavors that nourish both body and soul. May this collection be a constant companion on your path to wellness, offering not just sustenance but a celebration of the vibrant, delicious possibilities that a mindful, kidney-conscious diet can bring.

Here's to your health, happiness, and the joy of sipping toward a revitalized you.

Cheers!

www.ingramcontent.com/pod-product-compliance
Lightning Source LLC
Chambersburg PA
CBHW070720260726
48660CB00007B/2657